Simply Vegan: A Guide for Newbies and the Vegan Curious

Moniqua L. Sexton

Table of Contents

Introduction

My vegan journey started in 2012/2013. In 2012, I went to my gynecologist for my yearly women's exam. I expressed to her that I was having some digestive issues. I was only having a bowel movement once or twice a week, if that. I had severe gas buildup, meaning my stomach would bloat and ache with gas that I could feel in my shoulders and my back. I could not pass it unless I was laying down on my side, completely still for a long period of time. At this time, I was also having migraines. I'm talking about bed ridden migraines.

I had been on different medications and seen different doctors for my migraines and all they wanted to give me was medication. With my migraines worsening, having them a few times a week, and my digestive issues, I couldn't take it anymore. So, my gynecologist recommended I see a gastroenterologist. I went to see one and at first, he just wanted to give me medication. The medication didn't work and when I came back, the nurse was like, it usually doesn't work. He then suggested that I cut out red meat and stop consuming dairy because I may have an intolerance for it.

Cutting out red meat was no big deal. I was fine with chicken, turkey and fish. Dairy was a little harder because I loved cheese. My digestive issues improved. I was still having migraines. Over time, I slowly gave up chicken and then turkey. For a while, the only meat I would consume was fish. My digestive system began to work so much better. My migraines had subsided and became more spread out. But there was still something, like a feeling inside that I shouldn't be eating fish. This is around the time I started finding more vegans on Instagram.

After a while, I gave up fish, but I went back to consuming dairy and eggs. The thing is, I was becoming so nauseous after drinking milk or eating cheese. That was my body telling me to stop. By this point, my migraines had completely stopped. I was thankful for that.

The final straw for me was when I went on a college tour with my job at the time, with the kids from a local YMCA. All we had that weekend was pizza, donuts and more pizza. When I got home, I became so sick, that the next day, November 17, 2013, I was done with all animal products. I just couldn't do it anymore. It finally registered in my mind that consuming animal products was the root to my ailments.

This journey has taught me so many things and I have met so many amazing people. I feel alive, vibrant and energetic. I couldn't be happier. My body loves me for it and now. I have to say that health is the most important thing. You only get one body. Take care of it.

Reasons Most People Won't Go Vegan

- Fear of gaining weight

- Fear of losing weight

- Forming some sort of deficiency in vitamins, minerals and protein

- It's not the norm

- Fear of being isolated from friends and family

- Meat, dairy and eggs taste good

- God put animals on the earth for us to eat

- Plants feel pain too

- Animals would take over the world

- I'm allergic to gluten, soy and/or nuts

- I don't like salads

- It's how I was raised and what I am used to

I am not knocking any of these reasons as to not being vegan, in fact, a couple of these were my reasons to not being vegan in college when there were signs posted everywhere of animals being slaughtered. There was a vegan group on campus spreading awareness and I was a very ignorant college student. My reaction was, "I would never give up meat, that's just ridiculous." This is why I don't shame or judge those who have apprehensions about a plant based lifestyle.

I do want to give a little bit of information on each of these reasons. Many fear that they will gain or lose weight, and that really depends on what you are eating. There are a lot of unhealthy vegan foods on the market, some that are accidentally vegan, like Oreos. You can gain weight if you eat incorrectly and you can lose weight doing the same or not eating enough.

Deficiency seems to be the leading cause as to why people won't become vegan, specifically protein and B12. Well, let me ask you this question. Where do you think cows get their protein since they don't eat meat? What about gorillas and apes? They are all plant based animals and they are huge. They clearly have no protein deficiencies. As for B12, there are supplements but you can also get B12 from nutritional yeast, which I use in almost everything I cook. Two tablespoons contain 130% of your daily value. You can also get it from fortified nondairy milk. As for protein, you can get it from leafy greens such as kale, spinach and broccoli, as well as vegan protein powders, my favorite being Vega.

Being vegan to most seems intense or extreme because it is not something that is a part of the "norm" of society, though over recent years, more and more people have transitioned to a plant based lifestyle. The only thing I have to say to that is, why do you want to be accepted by people by being in the norm instead of doing what is best for you? No one else gives a shit about your health and no one can keep you healthy but you.

Many of us were not born vegan, and I will admit I am a tad jealous of those who were. I think my life would be totally different. Just because you were raised that way, does not mean that you have to continue to be that way. As you grow older, you become in charge of your own life and decisions, not your parents. You have the options of whether or not to consume animal products.

I know many people have this fear that they can't hang out with friends or family if they are vegan because restaurants don't cater to vegans. Well, as times are changing, many restaurants have vegan options or menu items that can be made vegan. Almost all restaurants have their menus online, so you can check ahead of time and you can call them and see which items can be customized to fit your dietary needs. It is bad business for restaurants to not cater to the dietary needs of each customer.

Meat, dairy and eggs taste good. Like the saying goes, "Just because its feels good, doesn't mean that it is good." This can also apply to food. Heart disease is the number one cause of death in America. Diabetes and obesity are increasing. Why? Animal products. Animals are not maintained like they used to be when our grandparents and great-grandparents were growing up. In those days, there was a such thing as cage-free and grass fed, because the animals actually did roam around on open land. Today, animals are repeatedly raped and inseminated to keep producing eggs and milk. Many are pumped with hormones and steroids to grow faster than they should. Everything controllers put in these animals, we are consuming. Times have changed drastically and I can't express that enough.

I've been seeing religion thrown around as a reason to not be vegan and that gets under my skin. People say God put animals on this earth for us to eat. Whether or not that is true, nowhere in the bible does God command us to eat animals. I will leave you with a few scriptures to read. Genesis 1:29-30 and Leviticus 11:1-47. People want to use the bible to justify not doing something, in Leviticus, it explicitly states that we are not to eat pigs because they are unclean. How many times do you see bacon across your television screen?

Plants feeling pain has to be the most ridiculous reason as to not be vegan. Plants do not bleed or cry out in pain like humans or animals do when being tortured or killed. That is an absurd idea. I am just being honest. It makes no sense.

Allergies to gluten, soy and/or nuts is very common among vegans and nonvegans alike. Many foods nowadays have gluten free versions and restaurants have gluten free items. There are also soy free ice creams, breads, yogurts and nondairy milk. As for nuts, just don't eat them. I think this goes for anyone actually, not just vegans. So this is another invalid excuse, but more of a common sense type of thing.

The stereotype that vegans only eat salads could not be further from the truth, and I will show you that later on in the book. Many foods that aren't vegan can be made vegan like macaroni and cheese, alfredo pasta, lasagna, spaghetti, tacos, burritos, burgers, you name it. There are vegan versions for almost everything. As an avid cook, I like getting creative in the kitchen.

I am not sure which of these reasons resonates with you, if any at all, but there is really no reason not to be vegan. If not for the animals or the planet, at least do it for yourself and your health.

Misconceptions about Vegans and Veganism

Vegans are looked at as these tree hugging, judgmental, crucifying, in-your-face types of people. I won't lie, there are some who are like that. Everyone has their own way of delivering the vegan message, I am not like that, which is why I wrote this guide. I want to help people who are newly vegan and those who want to go vegan, have an easy transition, and are able to stick with this lifestyle.

We say lifestyle because it's not a diet. Diets are temporary. Veganism is more than just about what you eat. It involves the clothes you wear and the products you use. There are many clothing, cosmetic and cleaning lines out there that are vegan and cruelty free.

Unlike some of my other fellow vegans who have high followings and tend to call nonvegans ignorant, unintelligent, weak-minded, uncompassionate, and other obscene and vulgar names, I welcome those who are curious and want to learn more. I welcome those who don't want to go vegan, but want to live a healthier life.

I think vegans and veganism gets a bad rep because of those individuals who use their platforms and their high followings as a way to demean those who are not vegan and steer those away who want to become vegan and that is not how all of us are. Majority of us are willing to help people step-by-step through the process of becoming vegan. These certain people also claim that you can't become vegan overnight, but don't give you ways to transition (which I will in the next chapter) and expect you to just be vegan.

We also get discriminated against as a whole in that we go around protesting and throwing paint on fur-wearers, creating havoc and mayhem at huge events. Believe it or not, many vegans are very peaceful people and only want to help better the planet and save the animals, in nonaggressive ways.

Veganism is about having compassion for the lives of all sentient beings and wanting to help sustain the planet that we live on, or we may all very well die out. It's about being healthy and living a lifestyle that is good for us and doesn't take the lives of innocent animals.

We are also not deficient in anything and if there are vegans that do have deficiencies, it's because they aren't eating enough and they aren't eating the right foods. I go to the doctor regularly and all of my levels are where they need to be, especially my protein and B12.

Please do not let the aggressive and hateful acts of some vegans, deter you from living a healthy life.

Tips on Transitioning to a Vegan Lifestyle

- One day a week being meatless (Meatless Monday)
- Reduce the meat you eat from every meal to maybe one or two meals a day, substituting the other meals with another form of protein like beans or lentils. Keep doing this until you aren't having any meat with your meals.
- Find a nondairy milk that you like and replace your dairy milk.
- If you love your scrambled eggs for breakfast, try tofu or chickpea scramble. I promise it is the best and you won't be packing in all the calories, cholesterol and fat, but you'll be getting more protein.
- Try different brands of vegan meat alternatives. Find ones that you like and stick with those.
- There are so many different brands of cheese alternatives and all are made with different bases (tapioca, nuts, tofu, etc.). Find one that you really like and use that instead of the dairy cheese. The vegan cheeses also come in your favorite flavors, so you won't be missing out.
- When you are ready, clean out your fridge and pantry, stocking it with only plant based food items. Always have fruits and veggies on hand

that you can grab quickly when you need to eat something or are on the go.

- Find vegan Meetup groups and go on vegan outings. Being vegan can sometimes seem lonely especially if you are the only one in your family and circle of friends. It makes it easier to be vegan when you have like-minded people around you.
- Become active in the vegan community on social media. There are so many vegans on Instagram and Pinterest. They are all very friendly and willing to help and welcome you with open emoji arms.
- If your friends and family aren't supportive, have a sit down and talk to them. Maybe even make them a vegan meal and/ or challenge them to see who can go the longest without eating meat.
- Educate yourself. Watch documentaries like *Food, Inc., Forks Over Knives, Cowspiracy, Earthlings, Fat, Sick and Nearly Dead, What the Health, Food Matters, Soul Food Junkies.*
- Find a local vegan co-op to volunteer at and get involved in the community to help spread the vegan message. It's a great way to meet more vegans and it will help you on your journey to hear their experiences.
- Don't try to become vegan overnight. It doesn't really work that way and if anyone tells you it does, they are lying. It is a process that takes patience, persistence, and faith.

Vegan/Raw Till 4/Raw Vegan

Many people don't know that when coming to a vegan lifestyle, there are different types of vegans. You have your regular vegan, which you can just be someone who doesn't consume animal products, but still eat a lot of vegan junk food, or a plant based vegan, which is what I identify with. Plant based vegans only consume foods that were grown from the ground, and they do not consume a lot of processed foods.

Raw till 4 vegans are those who only consume fruits and veggies in their raw form until 4 p.m. This consists of smoothies for breakfast, mono meals, and salads, basically anything that does not require any cooking. This particular lifestyle is highly publicized by some well-known vegans and I think that's the only reason that it's popular. I have tried this lifestyle many times and found that it just does not work for me. There are many days that I have eaten just fruit all day and then I have had something cooked for dinner, but it's been unintentional. Sometimes my body just craves fruit for majority of the day so that's what I do.

Raw vegans are those who only eat raw fruits and veggies, nuts and seeds. They don't eat anything cooked, period. This particular lifestyle is only led by a few, I know of one personally and she is very influential with the lifestyle. There are many apps and recipe books for raw foodists. I too have tried this lifestyle and am considering becoming 80% raw..

Now these are just my opinions. My suggestion is to try each lifestyle and see which one works best for you. Just because one lifestyle is highly publicized over the others, doesn't mean that it's better. Many people who are vegan, are plant based vegans, consuming cooked, whole, plant foods. There are not many people who led raw till 4 or raw vegan lifestyles, not saying that those lifestyles are bad, but because of social, personal, and logical reasons, many prefer plant based.

The reason none of the other lifestyles worked for me is because I love cooking. I took culinary arts in high school and I have always wanted to be a chef. Cooking makes me happy and on top of that, I am an exceptional baker, and I'm not just saying that. I love being in the kitchen, creating new meals and new desserts.

I do encourage that when you are starting on your vegan journey, that you try each of them out. With your current lifestyle or routine (work, kids, marriage, etc.), see which lifestyle would fit in. For someone who is always on the go, a raw vegan lifestyle may be best for you. It really just depends.

I must say, do not let all of these "famous vegans" influence your decision and make you feel that a particular lifestyle is the best lifestyle, and that if you can't succeed on that lifestyle, then there is something wrong with you and you are a bad person. That cannot be furthest from the truth. Also, these people are paid to advertise certain things and make certain types of videos. You have no idea what is going on when the cameras are off. You don't know their entire life so don't let them feed you stuff on a platter as truth. What works for some may not work for all. Remember that.

Also, this is your journey. You choose what is best for you and your life. No one else knows what will be best for you because they aren't living your life. All I am saying is, don't get caught up in all the hype. These people talk a good game, but at the end of the day, it's all about the money and what they can sell people.

Where Do Vegans Get Their Protein?

This is the number one question asked by nonvegans and instead of going on a tangent or rambling, I'll list a few ways we get our protein.

- Broccoli
- Kale
- Spinach
- Greens
- Vegan protein powders
- Oats
- Nuts
- Seeds
- Quinoa
- Beans
- Lentils
- Legumes
- Fruit
- Vegan protein bars
- Cabbage
- Cucumbers
- Cauliflower
- Tomatoes
- Mushrooms
- Avocado
- Figs
- Spirulina

- Hemp seeds
- Sweet potatoes
- Tofu
- Tempeh
- Seitan

As you can see, we vegans have no problem getting our protein and believe it or not, many of these plant foods have more protein per ounce than meat. Not only that, these foods have less calories, fat, sodium and cholesterol, and they didn't cost a life. It gets no better than that. So if you go vegan and people question your protein, ask them "Where do gorillas get their protein?"

Reasons to Cut Out Meat and Dairy

Americans consume on average 630 lbs of dairy each year. The article is a little outdated but I am sure the numbers have increased over the past 5 years. With that, Americans also consume 185 lbs of meat per year. These numbers are alarming, considering that this is per person, not as in a total. Do you know the effects that meat and dairy have on the brain and it's functions? No? Let me explain.

Dairy:

It's ironic that we are told that milk gives us calcium and builds strong bones, when in fact our bodies barely absorb any calcium and milk depletes bone mass. Also, before the advancement of technology, milk used to be drunk raw.

"Nowadays, milking cows are given antibiotics and most are also injected with a genetically engineered form of bovine growth hormone (rBGH). A man-made or synthetic hormone used to artificially increase milk production, rBGH also increases blood levels of the insulin-growth factor 1 (IGF-1) in those who drink it. And higher levels of IGF-1 are linked to several cancers."

If anything is linked to cancer, shouldn't that be an indicator to stop consuming it? Well, in this day and age, red flags tend to be ignored due to a person's own ignorant needs and wants. The most used excuse is because it tastes good, no matter any side effects. Did you know that 65% of people are lactose intolerant, and either don't know or don't care? This is especially important to know if you notice increased stomach pains and frequent constipation.

When I was younger, I stayed constipated to the point that I would rather die than to live through that pain and it only got worse as I got older. When I gave up dairy, that pain and constipation ceased to exist, leaving my mind free to be creative and not worry about stomach pains or how long to expect to be in the bathroom.

Here are **10 reasons to quit consuming dairy**:

1. **Ruins Skin**– Milk is a pro-inflammatory, meaning it could be making your acne worse, and if you don't have an acne problem, milk will certainly cause one. Consuming dairy makes your skin produce more sebum, which is clogging your pores and diminishing your complexion. Milk contains a great deal of the hormone IGF-1, which can make your acne spread and swell. Dairy has even been linked to eczema symptoms.
2. **Accelerates Aging**– Did you know that lactose is just sugar, sugar that most of us are intolerant of, and that sugar causes wrinkles? No? Well, now you do. The naturally occurring hormones in

milk age you, so imagine the damage the addition of more hormones and steroids can cause.

3. **Allergic Reactions**– Dairy allergy is one of the most common food allergies, with 12% of the US population being lactose intolerant. In children, whey and Casein are the most common allergies. Some think that these sensitivities wax and wane with age–I am here to tell you that that is not true. My symptoms of lactose intolerance got worse as I got older and I did continue to ignore them, until it became unbearable. Also, as a black or brown person, a good 70% of us are lactose intolerant because of how our DNA is made up.

4. **Highly Processed**– Unlike in the days of our grandparents and great-grandparents, cows are now fed antibiotics and shot up with hormones, and their milk is pasteurized, and homogenized.

5. **Fattening**– It is said that we should not drink our calories, yet we are constantly told to drink milk. Irony? I think so. Regardless of non-fat or low-fat, milk is calorically dense and adds hundreds of bad calories (yes, there's a such thing as bad calories). Milk also causes an insulin spike right after consumption, which can cause diabetes.

6. **Full of Pus**– Milking practices are disturbing. People like to think that milkmaids still milk cows. Sorry to burst your bubble, but cows are now milked in factories by giant machines, collecting not only milk, but scabs, pus and tears. In 2003 researchers found 298 million pus cells in a liter of California cow's milk.

7. **Hormones, Antibiotics and Misleading "Organic" Labeling**– Currently, companies do not have to tell you if they treat their cows with recombinant bovine growth hormone (rBGH). Cows treated with rBGH are more likely to suffer from mastitis and in turn be given antibiotics. Even scarier, just because something is labeled "organic" it might not be the case. That could just mean they are fed organic, yet are still pumped up with hormones and antibiotics.

Meat:

At many parties you see appetizers or snacks that's mainly meat and cheese. Of course, you dive in because it looks good and you know it tastes good. I used to be one of those people. Let me tell you, the stomachache later was not worth the indulgence. Many Americans consume meat for breakfast, lunch and dinner, as well as snacks (i.e. beef jerky and cheese, pork rinds, "lunch meat" which I am convinced is not even real meat). Do you know how much salt, fat, chemicals, hormones, and other unknown things, you and your family are consuming eating that much meat in a day?

According to the FDA, on average Americans are consuming 3,300 mg of salt per day. Do you know what foods are causing such high levels in sodium?

- breads and rolls – which we eat with everything. Switch out your normal bread with low sodium sprouted bread like Ezekiel or Genesis bread.

- luncheon meat, such as deli ham or turkey – like I said before, I don't even think it's real meat anyway. There are vegan options of deli meats that are much better.
- pizza – try making your own pizza with low sodium crust, sauce and ingredients. Try meat and cheese alternatives, or make a completely veggie pizza.
- poultry, fresh and processed—(Much of the raw chicken bought from a store has been injected with a sodium solution.) – just eliminate meat altogether
- soups – make your own or buy low sodium
- cheeseburgers and other sandwiches – use alternative meats or eliminate these altogether. You can always make your own veggie burgers from scratch.
- cheese, natural and processed – there is no such thing as natural cheese, given how it is made
- pasta dishes – use rice, quinoa, spelt, corn or amaranth noodles.
- meat dishes, such as meat loaf with gravy – replace the ground beef in meat loaf with black beans, lentils, mushrooms or even quinoa
- savory snack foods, such as potato chips, pretzels and popcorn – buy unsalted, kettle cooked or buy things like kale chips and seaweed.

Consume More Fruits and Veggies

The recommended serving of fruits and veggies is five. Five? Doesn't that seem rather low for foods that pack lots of nutrients and vitamins? What's funny is the food pyramid says to choose five fruits OR veggies, instead of AND. It also says to pick five fruits or veggies, but not how much of each. So what, two apples and three carrot sticks? Three leaves of kale and two grapes? You see my point here?

As you can see that meat is higher up on the food chain and it should be only eaten twice a day. If that is so, why do people eat it for every meal, between three and five times a day? It's funny how dairy is at the bottom of the pyramid as you should eat more of it than you do fruits or veggies.

Here's some facts on why you should consume more fruits and veggies:

1. They are easier for those who are on-the-go. Granted you properly clean them right after you buy them and store them in the fridge or in a basket, they are easy to pack. You can just grab whichever ones and go.
2. They make for great snacks, compared to chips, cookies, candy, etc. Most times people grab for the chips or any other unhealthy snacks because that is what is closest to them, or the only thing

they have in the house. Next time you go grocery shopping, don't buy the junk and instead buy a lot of fruits and veggies. You will notice the difference in how you feel.

3. They are okay to eat in numerous amounts. Have you ever heard of anyone going to the hospital for eating too many strawberries, or too much kale? No. You can eat as much fruit and veggies as you want and nothing will happen to you, other than you may be sitting on the toilet for a while, but that's never a bad thing.

4. You get in the most amount of nutrients and vitamins. I know almost every person in America takes some kind of vitamins for what they are lacking due to their poor diet. Many people don't even consume the recommended amount of fruits and veggies a day because they feel that they are too expensive. But wouldn't you rather spend a lot of money on something that will keep you out of the hospital and save you money long term? Think about your priorities.

5. They can be used to make anything. Many vegans buy fruits and veggies and make smoothies or juices. There are raw vegans who make all kinds of dishes out of them. Fruits and veggies don't have to just be fruits and veggies. For example, carrots, peppers, cucumbers and whatever other veggie you want, can be dipped in hummus, which is excellent by the way. I like to dip my apples in nut butter mixed with cinnamon. I think lack of knowledge and

creativity are why people don't consume a lot of fruits and veggies.

6. They are natural energy boosters, especially citrus fruits and leafy greens. They are packed with so many vitamins such as C and A, as well as fiber to keep you regular, and protein essential amino acids that your body needs. With that being said, drop the coffee and donuts, and grab some citrus fruits and leafy greens.

7. Having a rainbow (green, red, orange, yellow, blue and purple) plate of fruits and/or veggies, makes it more appetizing. For example, nutritionists recommend having every color of the rainbow on your plate. Not only is this for nutrient reasons but also because it looks more appetizing. If you have a pretty plate, you are more inclined to eat it. Eating by color will also lower your blood pressure and bad LDL cholesterol. This too can help you lose weight.

8. Last but not least, they just taste good. I know many fruits and veggies I didn't eat before I became vegan, I can't get enough of now.

When you have a healthy body by feeding it live food (meat is not live when it gets to the store and then on your plate), you are producing a healthy life.

Cook Your Own Food

There are numerous reasons to eat out less, stopping it all together if possible, and to cook your own food. I am only going to name a few of the important ones.

1. Food Poisoning. This is the most important reason. Anytime you eat out, you are saying that you are okay with the risk that you may contract food poisoning, or other foodborne illnesses like salmonella and E. Coli. You are taking these risks anytime you eat out especially at fast food restaurants, which are known to have bacteria everywhere. I used to work in a fast food restaurant (lasted three months) and I can tell you that they do not practice safety or sanitation measures 90 percent of the time. Many times that food has been sitting out, fallen on an unclean floor, touched by hands of persons who don't believe in washing them (which is how you can contract Hepatitis), amongst other things. I just want you to be aware that you are putting yourself at risk by letting a complete stranger prepare your food. Even if you're vegan, cross contamination and old food can give you food poisoning and anything else.
2. Saves Money. Do you know how much money you are really spending on your fast food bill? This also includes Starbucks. If you knew how much you spent in a year on fast food alone, you would be surprised. Take a look at your bank

statements and tell me how much you have spent already. Eating out really eats at your pocket.

3. Do you know what you're eating? That meat on your burger, do you even know where it came from? What about those ribs? Are you sure they came from a pig or a cow? Nowadays, meat farmers are not required to put where their meat comes from or if it's even really meat. It's not just the meat that may not be real, but also the cheese. To top it off, you don't know what is going into your food. Do you know what makes that food on your plate or in that bag taste good? Do you know if there is hair, spit, fecal matter, or bugs in it? Just because you can't see it, doesn't mean it isn't there or has been there. Half the time you won't know until it's too late.

4. Cooking food at home is fresher. When you prepare your meals yourself, you know that all of your ingredients are wholesome, fresh and you know what they are and where they came from, mind you if you follow a vegan diet. I cook a lot of plant based meals so I know that everything I prepared grew from the ground. All the herbs, spices, produce, everything. It's not only fresher, but it's healthier. You have more control of how much salt is in your food and you have the option of sea salt, which is the better option anyway.

5. Saves time. I always, always, always bring my lunch to work and that's mainly because I am a teacher. I can't really leave work to go anywhere. Even when I had a desk job, I brought my lunch. Many people only have 30 minutes for lunch and

if you are always buying it, you spend a good amount of that time either in a drive thru or standing in line, wasting your lunch. I prepare my lunches the night before so I can just grab and go in the morning. When lunch time comes, I can actually sit down and enjoy my lunch, not have to rush or scarf down my food.

These are the top reasons to stop eating out and prepare your own meals. Try it for a week and see what a difference it makes in your pocket and in your gut. Happy cooking!

Is Healthy Food Really Healthy?

You're walking down one of the food aisles and you see something bright colored out the corner of your eye. You turn to look and on the front of the box it says "All Natural". You pick it up and throw it in the basket. Then you keep walking and see something else that says "Fights Hunger". Throw that in the basket. You continue this until your basket is full of "healthy", "all natural", "hunger suppressant" foods. Are these foods actually what they claim to be?

Many times when we see these words on a box, we jump at the chance to buy it. We don't pay attention to the labels or nutrition facts. The ingredients are full of things that many of us cannot pronounce nor do we look them up to see what they are. We just see the big printed words on the front that states what is in the box is good for us.

Let's break down why these foods are not what they claim to be. So before you go and buy 20 boxes, packages or bottles, let's examine what is in the food or drinks. Many times aspartame, which is used as an alternative to sugar, is used in these foods. If you don't know what aspartame is, it is a chemical that is often used in rat poison and cigarettes.

Many chemicals like aspartame have addictive qualities, causing us to overeat things that are made to seem healthy. Also, many foods that have all of these chemicals, are topped with other ingredients that are disguised as healthy, such as vegetable oils, which include safflower, sunflower and other hydrogenated oils that are manmade.

Another thing to note is these "healthy" foods often times leave us still feeling hungry, causing us to overeat. This is led on by the addictive qualities. Now with fruits and vegetables, eating those until we are full is fine. But let's say we are eating "healthy" cookies, overeating those is not fine, causing us to become sick and consume a lot of fat.

Pricing for foods also contributes to how we buy foods. If something is marked as "healthy", 9 times out of 10, it has a huge sale tag on it with a price that seems reasonable. Of course we are going to opt to buy it; we're human.

Just because it says "healthy", "all natural" or whatever, doesn't mean it is. Look at the nutrition facts and the ingredients. See if there are any ingredients that are disguised as being healthy, and if you don't know, Google it. Google is your friend.

Organic v. Nonorganic

There is always a debate on whether or not you should buy organic or nonorganic. Many times it really just depends on where you live and whether organic options are readily available. I always say buy in season, because more than likely you will be able to purchase organic.

The main issue for those wanting to go vegan but can't because they feel organic is too expensive. If this is you, fear not, I am here to help. I personally buy organic as often as possible, and not just produce. I buy organic maple syrup, oats, frozen fruit and veggies, etc. If you do not have funds to buy organic fresh produce, buy it frozen. Just make sure that the ingredients read organic and that there is only fruit or vegetables and no preservatives or citric acid. Most times, you won't find any of that but you can never be too careful.

Another option would be to go to your local farmers market or your local farmer. They will be glad to give you some sort of discount and it's always cheaper and fresher. If you live somewhere that doesn't have a farmer's market look online to see if there are any co-ops or something similar. You always have options.

Whether or not organic or nonorganic is better, is really unclear. With farmers and companies now not being required to properly label their products or include everything that is in their products, you really can't tell. Now some fruits, like apples, you can tell which is organic and which is not. Nonorganic apples are very shiny, almost like they have been polished with wood shiner. You can also tell if produce is organic is if the five digit number on their label starts with a nine.

With other fruits and vegetables you can't really tell the difference between organic and nonorganic, so here is a list of the dirty dozen, plus some, produce that should be bought organic.

1. Apples

2. Strawberries

3. Grapes

4. Celery

5. Peaches

6. Spinach

7. Sweet bell peppers

8. Nectarines

9. Cucumbers

10. Cherry tomatoes

11. Potatoes

12. Hot peppers

13. Kale

14. Collard greens

15. Zucchini

16. Lettuce

17. Blueberries

These foods are typically high in pesticide residue, so it is always best, as possible, to buy these organic. Now foods that it doesn't matter whether or not you buy organic, include produce that we don't eat the outer skin.

1. Onions

2. Mangos

3. Sweet corn

4. Asparagus

5. Avocado

6. Pineapple

7. Papayas

8. Eggplant

9. Cantaloupe

10. Kiwi

11. Cabbage

12. Watermelon

13. Sweet potatoes

14. Mushrooms

15. Grapefruit

Most of these foods the pesticide is only on the outside, and doesn't get to the part that we actually eat. But make sure that you clean the outside very well before cutting into it because when you cut into it without cleaning it, the pesticide residue is on the knife and stays on it as you continue to cut your produce.

Reasons to Meal Prep

When I first became vegan, I was turned on to meal prepping. It was daunting at first because I saw so many photos on Instagram of people's after picks and they meal prepped for seven days, six meals a day, including snacks. It was very daunting and overwhelming. Then I realized that these people were vegan athletes. I wiped my brow in relaxation. I now meal prep for only five days a week, Monday thru Friday, which is when I work. I normally work 12 hours a day so I don't have time to come home or buy something even if I wanted to. Meal prepping has so many advantages, more than what I have listed. With being a new vegan, find certain meals that you like and don't mind eating every day. Stick with those at first and prep for the week. I promise you won't regret it.

- Saves money since you now have breakfast, lunch and dinner for the next few days, with some snacks thrown in there.
- You stick to your meals. When you have meals already prepared, you don't have to worry about what you're going to eat. If you're trying to lose weight (which I am definitely not), this helps because your meals are already portioned.
- Saves time to do other things. I don't mind cooking every day because I love to cook. But sometimes I don't have the time to and having meals already prepared saves time so I can do other more important things, like write this book.

- You know what you're eating. If you are one of those people who buys lunch every day at work and the local Chinese restaurant knows your name, where you work and your usual order because of so much take out, I can almost bet you don't know what's in your food. Preparing your own meals, you see everything that goes in it, unless you're a meat eater and an avid processed food in a box fanatic. Cook your own meals so you know what your body is intaking.
- If you plan your meals ahead of time, you won't have to go to the grocery store as much, and you won't spend so much money each trip on useless "food" that serves no nutritional purpose. You go in and get what you need to prepare your meals for the next few days, or if you're an overachiever, the entire week. (Don't be a show off.)
- Last thing, it's just an all-around good idea. Meal prep just keeps you on track with whichever of these goals you are trying to achieve.

With being a new vegan or wanting to go vegan, finding and/or making food can be hard if you are trying to make something every day. Maybe find two or three lunch or dinner recipes and switch them up each day, just so it doesn't get boring and like you're eating the same thing for lunch every day or dinner.

Snack Time Is Not Just For Kids

You remember snack time in elementary school? It was either after lunch or sometime in the morning. We always looked forward to snack time. If you didn't have snack time as a child, no worries. Many people today go long periods of time between meals, often feeling famished when it's time to eat, resulting in them eating any and everything in sight, mainly food that isn't good for them. This happens a lot of times with new vegans. Because you don't have snacks or vegan food readily available, you tend to grab whatever and not have second thoughts about it. Let's not do that.

Snack time is just as important as any other meal. I am the queen of snacks and I made an entire YouTube video on it. Snack time is very significant especially for a foodie. I have snacks in drawers in my bedroom, my purse and I pack snacks when I make my meals for the day. Snacks help to hold you over until you get your next meal. Snacks also help to keep you from binging when you do eat and keep you from feeling like you are going to pass out. People tend to be angry when they're hungry. Some snacks that you can buy are

- Fruit – mainly fruit that is easy to take on the go like berries, grapes, bananas, apples, oranges, etc.
- Seaweed – I love seaweed, the best thing since kale
- Veggie chips – I tend to only buy the ones that are actually made from vegetables and made with sea salt and either coconut or olive oil

- Nuts – any variety (this is only if you are not allergic)
- Graze – Graze snack boxes are great and you can make your own. There is even a setting to make sure that all snacks sent to you are vegan. For you free Graze box, you can use my code: 5CZXTWDFB
- Pretzels – and there are gluten free, low sodium pretzels, I buy them and they taste just as great.
- Clif Bars – one of my addictions and I like almost all flavors. These are also a really good source of protein
- Larabars – same as above
- Lightly salted popcorn or kettle corn – I prefer kettle corn because I love the sweetness but every now and again, I do get the lightly salted

There are many other healthy snack choices. I recommend 3-4 snacks a day, depending on your level of activity and how your meals are spread out.

Living Vegan on a Budget

So say you are a college student and you don't have a job, or you are living paycheck to paycheck trying to make ends meet. Whatever your situation, living vegan can be as cheap or as expensive as you make it. Vegan foods like faux meat and cheeses can be pretty pricey, so stick to the veggies, fruits, legumes, nuts and grains as possible. Rice and beans are very cheap to buy. If fresh fruit or veggies are not in your price range, like I said before, buy frozen, and I made a YouTube video on that as well.

This is also where meal prepping comes into play. Plan your meals for the week. Maybe on a Saturday or Sunday, set some time aside and plan meals. I will give some examples later on.

You also should plan your eating schedule and fit your snacks in there, this way when you go to the grocery store, you know exactly what to buy and how much. Many grocery stores, if you buy cases of any type of fruit or veggies, they give a discount. I once bought a 40 pound case of bananas for $18. That is not bad at all.

If you are eligible for food stamps, apply for food stamps, there is nothing wrong with that. When I was first vegan, I received $200 a month in food stamps and that was more than enough to survive since it's just me. Now that I have a better job and it pays more, I don't qualify but I am still able to afford my food. I keep myself on a strict food budget.

Eat what you have in the house before you go grocery shopping. Often times we spend money going grocery shopping when we have plenty of food in the pantry or fridge. That food sits there forever and then spoils. Try to only buy food that you are going to eat in that one week. Currently, my pantry and fridge looks bare because I only have food that I am going to eat during the week, then on the weekend, I restock with food for the next week.

If you are a college student, it is pretty easy to eat vegan, given that you have meal cards and can have all of your meals prepared. Try to stick to eating in the dining hall and not the restaurants on campus. This saves money on your dining card for the dining hall whenever you need it. Colleges are now offering healthier foods for students which is great, compared to when I was in college 6-10 years ago.

I know that you are allowed to take your meals to go, so while you are at it, take some fruit and veggies. You are already paying for it out of your tuition, why let it go to waste? Keep fruits and veggies in your room at all times. If you have a fridge in your room, stock up on produce. If not, just get enough to last you throughout the day and night when the dining hall closes.

When preparing your meals, try to find recipes that are suited for one person. This only applies to people who are single with no kids. I am not sure how to do this for couples or people with kids. Pinterest is the number one source of finding meals suited for one person, vegan and not. They also have great one dish meals, which are meals made using only one dish. This keeps the dishes down and the cost of food down since they don't require many ingredients.

When you go to the grocery store, always have a list and never go on an empty stomach. This a mistake that a lot of people make and then wonder why when they get to the register, their bill is north of $100. When you don't have a list, you tend to just pick up things. When you are hungry, your stomach tells you to buy what you're craving in that moment, and I can guarantee it isn't something healthy.

Eating Enough

A lot of times, new vegans fail at being vegan because they are always hungry and that stems from not knowing what to eat. Being on a vegan diet, you have to eat more than what you did when you were on the Standard American Diet (SAD). Vegan foods are much lower in calories, meaning that you have to eat more in order to get full.

When I first became vegan, I had this problem. I lost a lot of weight and I was tired and cranky all the time. I didn't know why, and though I did not revert back to meat eating, I did a little bit of research. I realized that my calorie intake was severely low and I was not eating nearly enough. At this time, I was also running 3-5 miles a day, burning more calories than I was eating.

So I ate more, a lot more, of plant based foods, often times going over 2,000 calories a day, but that was fine because I was active. There are many calculators online that tell you how many calories to eat per day. For me, at my height, weight and age and the amount of exercise I do a day, my calorie intake is 3,100. I never hit anywhere near that amount, but it's okay. As long as I hit 2,000, I'm good.

I don't exercise nearly as much as I used to because of my knees, but I still do yoga, and that is a total body workout, often times burning more calories than when I was running.

If you are someone who is very active, you have to eat way more than someone who doesn't exercise nearly as much. At minimum, a person's calorie intake must be 2,000 a day and honestly, if you are vegan, because plant based foods pass so quickly through our bodies, you have to eat much more than that.

So you are probably wondering how on earth you can eat more. Well, instead of half a cup of oats as recommended as a serving size, try eating 1 cup of oats. Instead of one plate or bowl of beans and rice, eat two. I would suggest eating twice as much as you would normally eat. I promise that you won't gain weight or feel sick. This only applies to eating plant based foods.

I know this may seem daunting at first, but after a while, it will be second nature. Your stomach is a muscle and it expands and contracts. You can train your stomach to hold as much food as possible, to where your stomach will be expecting a certain amount of food each time you eat.

I know this may be something tough to do for those coming to a vegan lifestyle from having an eating disorder, and though I don't know much if anything about eating disorders, I do know that a vegan lifestyle has healed many of their eating disorders. Most of these people are eating more than they have ever imagined. Yes, they sometimes do have reservations and thoughts of digression, but they keep pushing on. A vegan lifestyle allows you to be healthy and for your body to heal from years of abuse, neglect and damage. Eating disorder or not, we have all done some serious damage to our bodies and a vegan lifestyle is how we can heal it.

As a newbie or curious vegan, just know that you have to eat enough to get the amount of calories, vitamins, minerals and protein that your body needs. I know it may seem easier to get these things in on a meat eating diet, but think about the lives you will be saving, including your own. If we always took the easy way out, we would never know hard work or what it means to deserve something.

Staple Items

Dry Foods

- Rice
- Oats
- Quinoa
- lentils
- Millet
- Bulgur
- Beans (any kind)
- Non wheat pasta (rice, bean, quinoa, etc.)
- Flax seeds
- Chia seeds
- Nuts

Seasonings

- Thyme
- Oregano
- Parsley
- Rosemary
- Nutritional yeast
- Pink Himalayan Sea Salt
- Garlic powder
- Onion powder
- Mrs. Dash No Salt Seasonings (any kind)
- Fresh garlic

Produce

- Potatoes
- Broccoli
- Spinach
- Kale
- Mushrooms
- Carrots
- Greens
- Onions
- Grapes
- Berries (raspberries, blueberries, blackberries, strawberries, etc.)
- Bananas (got to have nana nice cream)
- Oranges
- Apples
- Pineapple
- Mango
- Watermelon
- Pears

Optional items

- Nut butters
- Pasta sauce
- Vegan alternative meats (Gardein, Beyond Meat and Field Roast are my favorite)
- Vegan cheese (Field Roast and Follow Your Heart are my favorites)
- Chips (I like veggie chips and kettle cooked)
- Unsweetened apple sauce (for baking)

- Nondairy milk (unless you make your own)
- Veggie burgers (there's too many brands that I like, and I also make my own)
- Vegan ice cream
- Vegan cookies
- Vegan yogurt

All of the produce items you can buy fresh or frozen, doesn't really matter. This isn't a complete list, it's just to get you started on building up your repertoire. I keep a lot of these in my house because I do a lot of cooking and often times use the same ingredients. I hope this has helped some of you. It's just the basics, but as you continue on this journey, you may find foods of your own that are staples for you.

Recommended Documentaries

- Forks Over Knives
- Cowspiracy
- Earthlings
- Food, INC
- Fat, Sick and Nearly Dead
- Vegucated
- Hungry for Change
- Plant Pure Nation
- Food Matters
- What the Health
- Soul Food Junkies
- Fed Up

Recommended Books

- The China Study
- Whole: Rethinking the Science of Nutrition
- Forks Over Knives The Cookbook
- The Lusty Vegan
- Thug Kitchen
- OhSheGlows
- The Happy Vegan
- The Food Revolution
- Vegan on the Cheap
- African Holistic Health
- By Any Greens Necessary
- Afro – Vegan

Recommended Brands

- Kiss My Face
- Jason Naturals
- Tom's of Maine
- Seventh Generation
- Dr. Bronner's
- Nature's Gate
- Crystal Body Deodorant
- EVOLVh
- Hugo Naturals
- Neal's Yard Remedies
- NatraCare
- NOW Foods
- Out of Africa
- Schmidt's Deodorant
- Trader Joe's Brand
- 365 (Whole Foods brand)
- Simple Truth (Kroger brand)

All of these brands are not just for women, they have men's products too. Yes, men, I would not think to exclude y'all!

How to Grocery Shop

Honestly, this goes for vegans and nonvegans alike. Whenever I go grocery shopping, I start in the produce section, meaning, I come in the store where the produce is. At all of my grocery stores, the produce section is always at the front, either on the left or right side of the store. It is always best to start there and fill up your cart with as much fresh fruit and vegetables as possible so that you don't fill it up with "other" stuff.

Another trick is to always get the small carts. This keeps you from piling stuff in. Once you have your fresh produce, you only have room left for things like grains, nuts, beans, pasta, and foods along those lines.

Always take reusable bags. When taking reusable bags, this means you can only get enough food to fit in those bags. You are restraining yourself from getting excess foods that you don't need. I normally take two to three bags in the store with me, even though I have several reusable bags in my car.

If your store has a healthy living section, that should be your next section once leaving the produce section. In the healthy living section of my grocery store is where I can buy bulk foods like nuts, oats, dry beans, rice quinoa, millet and make my own nut butter (yes, we have a nut grinding station).

After the healthy living section, then are the inner aisles where you find your pasta if that is not in your healthy living section. This is also where you can get your nut butters (if you don't have a nut grinding station), bread, crackers or whatever other types of foods or snacks you want to get. By this time, you don't really have room in your cart for a bunch of this stuff. In essence, you should be done grocery shopping.

Always keep these tips in mind when you go grocery shopping. This really helps to keep you from taking home foods that are not good for you and that you don't need. Saves you from buyer's remorse, and yes, that is a such thing even when grocery shopping.

If you need help finding health food items, ask an employee. It's their job to know where everything is and to help you find it.

Labels, Labels, Labels

Reading labels is super important when grocery shopping. Many packaged foods have milk and eggs in them these days, foods that can easily be made with nondairy milk and no eggs. A lot of vegans, even veterans (me included), have slipped and bought foods that had milk and eggs in them, not realizing it and then wondered why they became sick.

Not eating animal products for a long period of time and then eating them, can cause you to become sick because those foods became foreign to your body and your body rejects them, which is a good thing because animal products don't belong in your body to begin with.

Always read labels and if you don't have time to read labels, you can download an app called "Is It Vegan?" All you have to do is scan the barcode on the package and it will decipher the ingredients, letting you know if it's vegan or not. This was a lifesaver when I first became vegan because many packages have animal products in the ingredient list, disguised as something else.

Also, labels are important to read to see what kind of chemicals and other things that are being put into food. If there is an ingredient that you don't recognize or can't pronounce, your best bet is to not buy it. It is also good to get in the habit of googling ingredients that you don't recognize. If you don't recognize it, neither will your body and you don't want to risk becoming ill just because you didn't want to read the labels.

Companies are not forced to put all ingredients in a product on a label and they also aren't forced to be truthful about what's in the product. Don't you want to always know what you're putting in your body? I would suggest staying away from processed packaged foods. If you can make it yourself, do so, or buy packaged foods that aren't heavily processed and that you know what every ingredient is.

Recipes

The next 20+ pages are filled with recipe ideas for breakfast, lunch, dinner and dessert. They all consist of ingredients that are easy to find and easy on the pockets. Any recipe can be made gluten free with a few tweaks and if you don't like soy or it doesn't agree with your body, exclude that ingredient. Make these recipes your own and to your liking.

I love cooking and each one of these recipes was made with love, creativity, and a hungry stomach. Many were made by just opening the pantry and fridge, and just grabbing stuff. It all turned out well. Some I did have to adjust the ingredients, but that is something you learn when making vegan food. Spices and herbs are important. Figure out which ones you like that go great together.

Protein Pancakes

1 ½ c all-purpose wheat flour (use oat flour if you are gluten intolerant)

2 tbsp. Peanut Butter and Co Cinnamon raisin swirl peanut butter (any nut butter is fine)

2 tbsp. flax meal + 6tbsp. water

1 c nut milk

Optional:

Fruit of your choice

Blend all the ingredients in the blender to desired consistency. Heat nonstick pan and pour in batter to desired size. I topped these with more flax seeds for omega fatty acids and fiber as well as raspberries and organic maple syrup.

Mug Cake

5 tbsp. oat flour (if you don't have any, process some oats, that's what I did)

1 1/2 tbsp. cacao powder

1 tbsp. agave nectar

1/4 tsp vanilla extract

4 tbsp. hemp milk (or any vegan milk of your choice)

1 tsp coconut oil (olive oil works fine too)

2 tbsp. of water

Mix ingredients and pour into a coffee mug or small glass bowl (that's microwave safe), and microwave for two minutes. Enjoy!

Overnight Oats

1 cups rolled oats

1 ½ c almond milk

¼ c chia seeds

1-2 tsps. of cinnamon

2 tbsp. of coconut sugar

      Pour all ingredients in a mason jar and mix well. I chose a 30 oz. mason jar because I knew I would add a copious amount of toppings. Cover and let sit in the fridge overnight. In the morning you can add whatever toppings you like. I chose muesli, hazelnuts, frozen blueberries and organic maple syrup.

Peanut Butter Protein Balls

½ c crunchy peanut butter

½ c oats

¼ c pure maple syrup

1 tbsp. chia seeds

1 tbsp. flax seeds

½ unsweetened dark chocolate chips

Mix all ingredients in a bowl, well. Take a tablespoon and roll into a ball. Coat with chia and flax seeds. Do this until all of the mixture is done. Place balls into a container and cover, placing in the refrigerator for 30 minutes or overnight, until firm.

Bean Loaf

Ingredients:

2 cans of organic beans (I used garbanzo and tri bean blend)

1 tbsp. minced garlic

1 tsp oil (I used grapeseed)

1 c whole wheat flour (or your choice)

1 c organic marinara sauce

1 c diced bell peppers (yellow, orange and red, green if you want)

2 handfuls of bite size pretzels, broken

2 tsp basil

2 tsp sage

2 tsp lemon pepper seasoning

2 tsp thyme

Preheat oven to 350F. Place all ingredients in a food processor, or blender that has a pulse setting. Pulse until it becomes the same consistency as ground meatloaf. Place in a nonstick loaf pan and top with organic ketchup, then bake for 30-45 minutes, until browned.

I normally pair this with rice or mac n "cheeze", and some sort of veggie. I used avocado here because it has good fats and mixing these together has a great taste. Depending on what sides you choose, this can be lunch or dinner.

Quinoa and Bulgur Kale Salad

1 c quinoa and bulgur mix

2 tbsp. Sunflower seeds

1/2 c and 2 tbsp of olive oil

1/2 c dried cranberries

1/2 small onion

4 c of kale leaves, torn into small pieces

2 tbsp fresh lemon juice

Himalayan sea salt

Cook quinoa and bulgur as usual. Sauté onions, sunflower seeds and dried cranberries in the 2 tbsp of olive oil.

In a food processor, take 2/3 of the kale and the lemon juice and pulse until chopped. Slowly pour in the 1/2 c of olive oil.

Get a large bowl and pour in quinoa, onion mix and kale pesto. Mix well, adding sea salt to taste. Presto!

Vegan Chili

1/2 large purple onion, diced

1 1/2 cans black beans, rinsed and drained

1 pck of Beyond Meat meatless ground (I used the feisty flavor)
2 c water

2 c vegetable broth

1 c black rice

1/2 red bell pepper

1/2 yellow bell pepper

1/2 green bell pepper

2-4 tbsp. chili powder (depends on your taste)

Boil water then add rice. Cook until water is almost gone.
Sauté meatless ground, bell peppers and onions until onions are clear. Add black beans and rice. Pour in vegetable broth and add chili powder. Simmer until hot, about 20 min. Enjoy!!

"Beef" Stew

2 cans black beans, rinsed and drained

1 c black rice, optional

2 c water

1 tbsp. Earth Balance Original buttery spread

6 medium red potatoes, diced

thyme

basil

chili powder

vegetable broth

1 pck of Beyond Meat Beefless Ground, fiesty flavor

Boil the two cups of water for the rice. In a pot, sauté potatoes in butter until soft. Add in Beyond Meat beefless ground (feisty flavor). Cover and cook until it is all thoroughly cooked. Add in black beans and cooked rice. Add all seasonings and vegetable broth. I usually measure with my eyes for the broth. It really just depends on how thin or thick you want it to be.

Lentil Loaf

2 cups water

1 cup green lentils

2 tbsp. ground flaxseeds + 4 Tbs water

1/2 white onion, diced

1 tsp. olive oil

1 c rolled oats

1 c tomato sauce (I used spaghetti sauce)

1 tsp. garlic powder

1 tsp. dried basil

1 tsp. dried parsley

1/2 tsp. salt

1/4 tsp. black pepper

1/4 c BBQ sauce (any kind)

2 tbsp. ketchup

Bring water to a boil. Add lentils and simmer 25 – 30 minutes, until water is evaporated. Drain any excess water and partially mash lentils. Put into a mixing bowl and let cool just a bit.

Mix the flaxseeds and water and let sit for about 15 minutes.

Sauté the onion and bell peppers in the oil over medium heat. Cook for until the onion is translucent.

Stir the onion and oats into the lentils until mixed. Add the flax mixture, tomato sauce, garlic, basil, parsley, salt, and pepper. Mix well.

Spoon into loaf into nonstick pan. Smooth the top with the back of a spoon. Top with the BBQ sauce and ketchup.
Bake at 350 degrees for about 45 minutes until the top of the loaf is dry, firm, and golden brown. Let cool in pan for about 10 minutes. Run a sharp knife around the edges of pan then turn out onto a serving platter. Top with ketchup if needed.

Quinoa Bowl w/ Hummus Dressing

2 c. fresh/frozen broccoli florets

2 c. fresh spinach, chopped

1 ripe avocado

1 c. quinoa, your choice in color

2 c. water

Pink Himalayan Sea Salt, to taste

Hummus Goddess Hummus Dressing

Directions:

Cook quinoa in water. Once done, let cool.

Steam broccoli and add spinach when broccoli is almost to desired consistency.

Mix quinoa with veggies in a bowl, adding salt. Top with avocado and hummus dressing.

Zesty Ranch Portobello Steak Dinner

4 Portobello mushrooms

1/4 c vegan zesty ranch salad dressing & marinade

Directions:

Wash and marinate mushrooms. Let them sit for about 20 min in the fridge. When you are almost ready to cook them, heat up the grill. I used a George Foreman grill, so I do not have a time for how long they should cook.

Mashed Potatoes:

1 bag small red potatoes

1/2 c Nondairy Milk

1/4 c vegan sour cream (Sour Supreme)

3 stalks green onions, chopped

Pink Himalayan sea salt to taste

1 tbsp. vegan butter

Directions:

Wash and then boil potatoes. Once they are mashable (test with a fork), drain the water and then mash them. Add in all other ingredients. The measurement for the milk can be more or less based on your desired creaminess. I also left the skin on my potatoes because the skin has vitamins and nutrients. Plus, it adds color.

Fried Cabbage:

1/2 head of purple cabbage, chopped

1 white onion, chopped

sea salt to taste

Oil to fry in (your choice, I used avocado oil

Directions:

Heat a pot or skillet with your choice of oil. Once hot, put in cabbage and onion, covering with a lid. Let fry for about 20-30 min., or until cabbage is somewhat translucent.

Mushroom Stuffed Collard Greens

1 tbsp. oil (your choice)

1 tbsp. vegan butter (I used Smart Balance with flaxseed oil)

1 can diced tomatoes

2 c. low sodium vegetable broth

1 onion, grated or finely chopped

8 large collard greens leaves, stems removed

2 c. chopped mushrooms (your choice)

1/2 c. cooked rice or quinoa

Zest of 1 lemon

2 tsp. paprika

1/2 tsp. dill seeds

Salt and pepper, to taste

Directions:

Heat oil and butter in skillet. Add tomatoes, veggie stock, and onion, all but 2 tbsp. Add salt and pepper. Once mixture is boiling, reduce heat and let simmer. Now prepare your greens and stuffing.

Blanch leaves for 1-2 min. in boiling water. Drain, rinse with cold water and pat dry.

Sauté mushrooms until soft. Mix mushrooms, rice/quinoa, paprika, dill seeds and lemon zest with remaining 2 tbsp. of onion. Add 3/4 tsp. salt and 1/4 tsp. pepper. Divide mixture among the leaves. Fold bottom edge and sides then roll up the leaves.

Place the stuffed greens seam down in sauce. Cover and simmer on low for 30-45 min. Once done, you can pair it with any side you choose.

Mexican Dip

1 tbsp. olive oil

1 onion, chopped

2 cloves of garlic

1 c brown rice

1 tsp paprika

2 c vegetable broth

¼ tsp of black pepper

4 roma tomatoes

2 cans pinto beans, rinsed and drained

1 can mild dice green chile salsa

1 cup corn

1 pck of Daiya cheddar cheese

Preheat oven to 350F. Lightly grease a 9 x 13 pan or use a nonstick pan, and set aside.

In a sauce pan, heat oil and sauté onions until soft and then add garlic. Add rice, paprika and vegetable broth. Add pepper and let simmer for about 20 minutes. Once done, pour into pan and stir in the remaining ingredients. Cover with foil and bake for 45 minutes. After that, remove from oven, add cheeze and then bake until cheese is melted. Let cool and enjoy as a meal itself or put it on some tortilla chips.

Cauliflower Crust Pizza

1 whole cauliflower head

1/2 c unsweetened apple sauce

1/4 tsp Italian seasoning

1/4 tsp onion powder

1/2 c vegan Parmesan cheese

Salt and pepper to taste.

Process cauliflower until chopped finely. Microwave for five minutes. Let cool. Pour onto towel or paper towel and squeeze out excess water. Put into a bowl and mix in all other ingredients. Spread to your desired shape crust. Bake in preheated oven of 400F for 40 min. Add toppings and bake at 450F for 8 minutes or until toppings look done.

My toppings are chunky mushroom tomato sauce, spinach, fresh tomatoes and Daiya mozzarella flavored vegan cheese.

Coconut Sesame Fried Rice

1 c rice w/ wild rice

1 c quinoa

Sesame oil

Soy sauce

1 pck frozen peas

Shredded carrots

Coconut flakes

Cook rice and quinoa together normally. Heat a pan and add in carrots, peas and coconut flakes in a little bit of oil. Add in rice and when it's almost done, drizzle on some sesame oil and soy sauce.

"Beef" and Chili Verde

1 pkg Beyond Meat Ground Crumbles

1 large red bell pepper, chopped

1 large onion (red or yellow), chopped

6 cloves garlic, chopped

1 tbsp. chili powder

2 tsp. ground cumin

1/4 tsp. cayenne pepper, or to taste

1 16-ounce jar green salsa, green enchilada sauce or

taco sauce

1/4 c water

1 15-oz can pinto or kidney beans, rinsed

1 small can of mushrooms (optional. I just really love

mushrooms)

Eat with:
Rice (I prefer Basmati rice) or blue/white corn tortilla
chips

Cook veggie protein, bell pepper and onion in a large
saucepan over medium heat, crumbling the meat with a
wooden spoon, until the meat is browned, 8 to 10

minutes. Add garlic, chili powder, cumin and cayenne; cook until fragrant, about 15 seconds. Stir in salsa (or sauce) and water; bring to a simmer. Reduce heat to medium-low, cover and cook, stirring occasionally, until the vegetables are tender, 10 to 15 minutes. Stir in beans and cook until heated through, about 1 minute.

Mushroom Stuffed Cabbage

Ingredients:

1 tbs grapeseed oil

1 tbs Smart Balance butter

1/2 jar Amy's salsa

2 tomatoes, diced

2 c vegetable stock

1 onion, grated or minced

6-8 cabbage leaves

8oz pack of mushrooms, pulsed

1/2 c cooked rice, any kind

Grated zest of a lemon

2 tsp paprika

1 tsp pink himalayan sea salt

1 tsp black pepper

1 tbs flax seeds, 3 tbs water

Directions:
Combine flaxseed + water in small container to make
flax egg. Set aside.

Heat oil and butter in skillet. Add salsa, tomatoes, vegetable stock and onions.
Simmer gently.
Bring a large pot to boil to blanche cabbage leaves to desired softness.
Combine the rest of the ingredients (mushrooms, rice, lemon zest, seasonings, and flax egg) in a large bowl.
Spoon mixture into leaves. Fold over sides and edges.
Place folded side down in sauce.
Simmer for 30-45 min.
Serve.

Vegan Philly Cheesesteak

Ingredients:

2 bell peppers, any color, sliced

1 onion, sliced

2-4 portobello mushrooms, sliced

1 can green chilies

2 tbsp nutritional yeast

1/2 tsp pink himalayan sea salt

Dash of pepper

Dash of cayenne pepper

Hoagie buns

4 slices of vegan cheese, i used Field Roast chao cheese

coconut herb

Directions:
Slice all of your veggies and mushrooms and saute them
to your liking. Add in spices. Top with 4 slices cheese,
cook until melted.
Slice your hoagie bun down the middle or scoop out the
middle. Add your filling, and pair with chips or your
choice of side.

French Toast

Ingredients:

1 c. Nondairy milk

1 tbs. flax meal

1 tsp. vanilla

1 tsp. cinnamon

2 c. of your favorite fruit, chopped if needed

4 pieces of vegan bread

Pure maple syrup

Directions:

Mix all ingredients in a bowl except for fruit and syrup, then let sit.

Grease and heat a skillet.

Coat both sides of bread with mix. Please be sure to not soak bread in mixture. If need be, brush the bread on both sides with mix.

In the hot skillet, place your bread and cook for 2-3 min., or until golden brown, then flip. Do this until all pieces of bread are done.

Plate, rope with fruit and syrup, pour a glass of fresh OJ and enjoy!

Coconut Pumpkin Seed Banana Bread

3 very ripe bananas

1/3 c of organic coconut sugar

3 ½ tsp baking powder

1 ½ c oats, processed into a flour consistency (or use oat flour)

Handful of shredded coconut

Handful of pumpkin seeds

½ c coconut oil

½ tsp nutmeg

1 tsp cinnamon

Preheat oven to 350F.

Mash bananas and mix with coconut sugar, coconut oil nutmeg and cinnamon, mix well. Make sure there are no lumps. Fold in shredded coconut and pumpkin seeds (or you can use nuts). Pour in a greased bread pan, sprinkling coconut and seeds (or nuts) on top. Bake for 30-40 minutes. Let cool for about 10-15 minutes.

Cranberry Orange Oatmeal Raisin Biscuits

2 cups flour

1 tablespoon orange zest (about 2 oranges)

1 teaspoon baking powder

1/2 teaspoon salt

1 cup unrefined sugar (or equivalent of other sweetener)

1/3 cup unsweetened applesauce

1/2 cup olive oil

1/3 cup fresh orange juice

1 teaspoon vanilla extract

2/3 cup raisins and dried cranberries

Quick oats

Directions

Preheat oven to 350 degrees. Lightly oil a cookie sheet or use wax paper.

In a medium bowl, combine flour, orange zest, baking soda and salt. Set aside.

In a separate bowl mix sugar, applesauce and olive oil. Add vanilla and orange juice and blend well.

Pour the wet mixture into the dry mixture, and combine. Stir in quick oats. I didn't measure them. I sprinkled them in to my liking since I love oats.

Drop dough onto your prepared sheet, and bake for 15–20 minutes. Let cool on sheet for 5 minutes before transferring to a wire cooling rack.

Use fresh orange juice to achieve optimum flavor. I juiced the oranges in my juicer, but if you don't have a juicer, you can always hand squeeze them.

For extra texture, add some nuts such as almonds, walnuts, or pecans.

Meal Plan

This meal plan is to guide you on what a week of eating may look like. You can also check my YouTube channel for what I eat in a day. You can feel free to deviate, change things, add or eliminate. This is not a strict follow the book kind of thing.

Monday

Breakfast:

Overnight oats (see recipe pg. 60)

1 glass orange juice

Snack:

Handful of nuts

Lunch:

Quinoa Bulgur Kale Salad (see recipe pg. 64)

Snack:

1 cup of fruit, your choice

Dinner:

Zesty Ranch Portobello Dinner (see recipe, pg. 70)

Tuesday

Breakfast:

Green Smoothie (kale, banana, pineapple and avocado)

Snack:

Non dairy yogurt and fruit or granola

Lunch:

Zesty Ranch Portobello Dinner (leftovers from last night)

Snack:

Hummus and carrot chips

Dinner:

Mexican Dip (see recipe, pg. 74)

Wednesday

Breakfast:

French toast (see recipe, pg. 80)

1 glass orange juice

Snack:

Fruit of your choice

Lunch:

Mexican Dip (leftovers from last night)

Snack:

Snack size bag of popcorn (of course without butter)

Dinner:

Coconut Sesame Fried Rice (see recipe, pg. 77)

Thursday

Breakfast:

Peanut Butter Protein Balls (see recipe, pg. 61)

Snack:

Seaweed or kale chips

Lunch:

Coconut Sesame Fried Rice (leftovers from last night)

Snack:

Fruit and nuts

Dinner:

Mushroom Stuffed Collard Greens (see recipe, pg.72)

Friday

Breakfast:

Leftover Peanut Butter Protein Balls

Snack:

Non dairy yogurt and granola

Lunch:

Mushroom Stuffed Collard Greens (leftovers from last night)

Snack:

Your Choice

Dinner:

Quinoa Bowl w/ Hummus Dressing (see recipe, pg. 69)

Saturday and Sunday

You can eat whatever you have left over from the week. I did not include desserts because that is not typically part of a meal plan, but if you want desserts, feel free to add them. This was just a sample meal plan, to give you an idea if what I eat in a typical day. Of course, I only drink water or tea, which is why I did not add any drinks. Do not feel that this is such a strict plan. I don't want you to feel like this is how you have to eat all the time. Change it up if you want. Of course all of my recipes are fresh and made from scratch. I used to love food that came in boxes that were easy to prepare, but just because it's vegan, doesn't mean it's good for you.

Sources

The Average American Ate a Ton This Year – npr.org

Osteoporosis Milk Myth – saveourbones.com

How Many Pus Cells Are In Your Milk – foodmatters.tv

Recombinant Bovine Growth Hormone – cancer.org

Lactose Intolerance – ghr.nlm.nih.gov

Milk consumption: aggravating factor of acne and promoter of chronic diseases of Western societies – ncbi.nlm.nih.gov

Meat and Cheese may be as bad for you as smoking – sciencedaily.com

Pasteurized milk 150 times more contaminated with blood, pus and feces than fresh milk - videos the CDC won't show you – naturalnews.com

Author Info

Twitter: @blackvegnauthor

Facebook/YouTube: The Black Vegan Author

Pinterest: @theblackveganauthor

Instagram: @theblackveganauthor

Email: moniquasexton@me.com

Website: www.theblackveganauthor.com